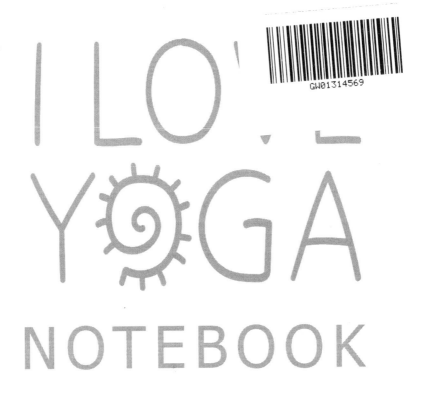

I LOVE YOGA NOTEBOOK

With Motivational, Inspirational & Funny Yoga Quotes

This Notebook Belongs To:

E-mail:

Phone:

GOALS:

Accomplishments:

Habit Tracker	1	2	3	4	5	6	7	8	9	10

Appointments & Special Dates:

Yoga is not to be performed. Yoga is to be lived.

Breathe. Believe. Receive.

In stillness all conflict must end. - Phillip Urso

Even after you've rolled up your mat, yoga continues. - Zubin Atré

Yoga is the perfect opportunity to be curious about who you are.
- Jason Crandell

Even after you've rolled up your mat, yoga continues. - Zubin Atré

Practice love until you remember that you are love.
- Swami Sai Premananda

Compassion is the religion of the heart. - Ma Jaya Sati Bhagavati

Everyone can do Ashtanga. Except lazy people. - Sharath Jois

In the darkness, I am light.

Yoga is the process of eliminating pain – pain form the body, mind and the society. - Amit Ray

Never underestimate a woman with a yoga mat.

Yoga does not change the way we see things. It transforms the person who sees. - B.K.S. Iyengar

Yoga is the perfect opportunity to be curious about who you are.
- Jason Crandell

The more we sweat in peace the less we bleed in war.
- Vijaya Lakshmi Pandit

Please grant me coffee to change the things I can and yoga to accept the things I can't.

Don't forget to breathe!

Submit to a daily practice. Your loyalty to that is a ring at the door. Keep knocking, and eventually the joy inside will look out to see who is there.

Yoga is not about self improvement. It's about self acceptance.

One becomes firmly established in practice only after attending to it for a long time, without interruption and with an attitude of devotion.

You cannot do yoga. Yoga is your natural state. What you can do are yoga exercises, which may reveal to you where you are resisting your natural state. - Sharon Gannon

Quiet the mind and the soul will speak.

I don't trust anyone who doesn't like yoga, pizza, or puppies.

When you inhale, you are taking the strength from God. When you exhale, it represents the service you are giving to the world.

- B.K.S. Iyengar

First month paining, second month tired, third month flying.
- Sharath Jois

Yoga is a journey toward your inner core to find your inner bliss.
- Debasish Mridha

I have been a seeker and I still am, but I stopped asking the books and the stars. I started listening to the teaching of my Soul.

- Rumi

Make an attitude to be in gratitude, you will find the whole Universe will come to you. - Yogi Bhajan

The more you listen to your breath, the more you can hear the voice of your soul. - Ma Jaya Sati Bhagavati

Sometimes you have to let go to be free.

Have only love in your heart for others. The more you see the good in them, the more you will establish good in yourself.
- Paramahansa Yogananda

Wisdom is knowing we are all One. Love is what it feels like and Compassion is what it acts like. - Ethan Walker III

The attitude of gratitude is the highest yoga. - Yogi Bhajan

It takes a lot of courage to be happy. - Ma Jaya Sati Bhagavati

Do your practice and all is coming. - Sri K Patthabi Jois

Yoga takes you into the present moment, the only place where life exists.

The most important pieces of equipment you need for doing yoga are your body and your mind. - Rodney Yee

Sometimes you have to let go to be free.

Stirum sukham asanam. Seated posture should be steady and comfortable.

Yoga is not about self improvement. It's about self acceptance.

When you own your breath, nobody can steal your peace.

I got 99 problems and I'm gonna go to yoga and solve about 53 of them.

It is not arrogant or egotistical to feel good inside. You had nothing to do with it. It's simply the honest response to clearly perceived Reality. - Erich Schiffman

Your task is not to seek for love, but merely to seek and find all the barriers within yourself that you have built. - Rumi

Let your practice be a celebration of life - Seido lee deBarros

Inhale, and God approaches you. Hold the inhalation, and God remains with you. Exhale, and you approach God. Hold the exhalation, and surrender to God. - Krishnamacharya

A photographer gets people to pose for him. A yoga instructor gets people to pose for themselves. - Jay Fields

The most important pieces of equipment you need for doing yoga are your body and your mind. - Rodney Yee

Yoga means addition - addition of energy, strength and beauty to body, mind and soul. - Amit Ray

Nothing can bring you peace but yourself.

Eye on the drishti!

Monday. Nothing a bit of Yoga can't fix.

Yoga is a method to come to a nondreaming mind. Yoga is the science to be in the here and now. - Osho

Practice and all is coming. - Sri K. Pattabhi Jois

Yoga teaches us to cure what need not be endured and to endure what cannot be cured. - Geeta Iyengar

Just breathe.

Sky above. Earth below. Peace within.

Yoga is the journey of the self, through the self, to the self.
- The Bhagvad Gita

You must be the change you wish to see in the world. - Gandhi

Desire, ask, believe, receive. - Stella Terrill Mann

Yoga is the journey of the self, through the self, to the self.
- The Bhagvad Gita

You cannot always control what goes on outside. But you can always control what goes on inside.

To find inner bliss and happiness through yoga, learn to accept things as they are by changing your thoughts. - Debasish Mridha

Yoga is not to be performed. Yoga is to be lived.

Yoga is not for the flexible. It's for the willing.

Quiet the mind and the soul will speak.

Mindfulness helps you go home to the present. And every time you go there and recognize a condition of happiness that you have, happiness comes. - Thich Nhat Hanh

Give this world good energy.

Get the inside right. The outside will fall into place. - Eckhart Tolle

Remember the emphasis on the heart. The mind lives in doubt and the heart lives in trust. When you trust, suddenly you become centered. - Osho

Be at least as interested in what goes on inside you as what happens outside. If you get the inside right, the outside will fall into place. - Eckhart Tolle

Trust the vibes you get. Energy doesn't lie.

Breathe. Believe. Receive.

For me, yoga is not just a workout – it's about working on yourself.
- Mary Glover

When we can remove the masks of our own making, then the one who has been longing to be seen sees itself unbounded, just as it is.

Ashtanga yoga is 99 percent practice, one percent theory.
- Sri K. Pattabhi Jois

The rhythm of the body, the melody of the mind & the harmony of the soul create the symphony of life. - B.K.S. Iyengar

Yoga will always be transformational, even when it stops being cool. - Victoria Moran

To perform every action artfully is yoga. - Swami Kripalu

Embrace messy hair and yoga pants.

Yoga teaches us to cure what need not be endured and to endure what cannot be cured. - Geeta Iyengar

A flower does not think of competing with the flower next to it. It just blooms.

Vibration is the core of the spirit. It is the breath of life.
- Suzy Kassem

Breathe through it, and release anything that does not serve you.

Anybody can breathe. Therefore anybody can practice yoga.

The world is the gymnasium where we come to make ourselves strong. - Swami Vivekananda

Yoga is the art work of awareness on the canvas of body, mind, and soul. - Amit Ray

Be the energy you want to attract.

When you find peace within yourself, you become the kind of person who can live at peace with others. - Peace Pilgrim

Get out of yourhead and into your heart. Think less, feel more.
- Osho

Yoga is not about touching your toes. It is what you learn on the way down. - Jigar Gor

Practice love until you remember that you are love.
- Swami Sai Premananda

True meditation is about being fully present with everything that is--including discomfort and challenges. It is not an escape from life.
- Craig Hamilton

Blessed are the flexible, for they shall not be bent out of shape.

He shining, everything shines through him. - Bhagavad Gita

The pose begins when you want to leave it.

Remember, it doesn't matter how deep into a posture you go – what does matter is who you are when you get there. - Max Strom

I am centered. I am balanced. I am at peace.

The wisdom obtained in the higher states of consciousness is different from that obtained by inference and testimony as it refers to particulars.

Healthy plants and trees yield abundant flowers and fruits. Similarly, from a healthy person, smiles and happiness shine forth like the rays of the sun. - B.K. S Iyengar

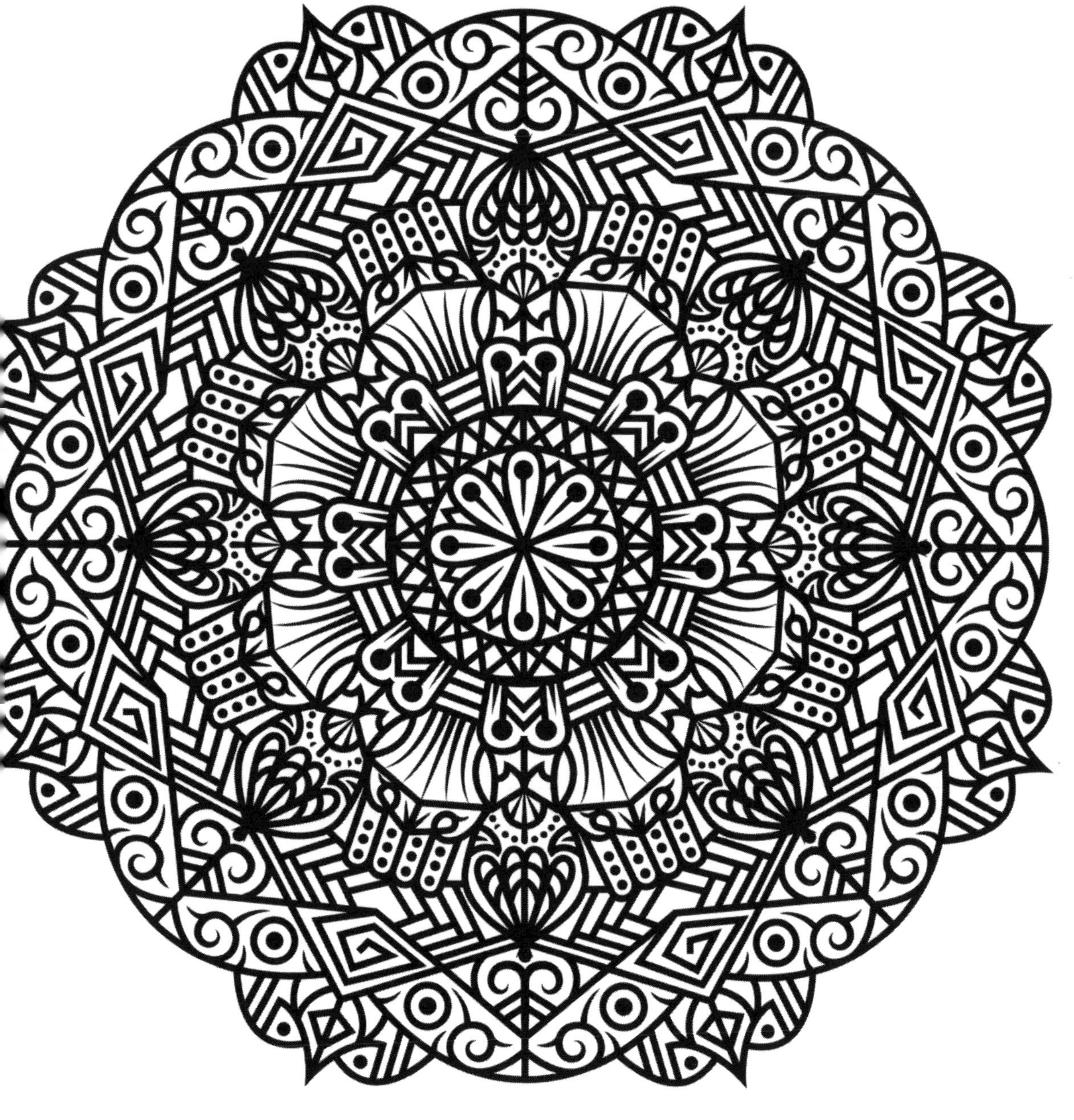

Bonus Mandala Adult Coloring Book Page

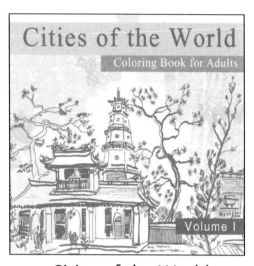

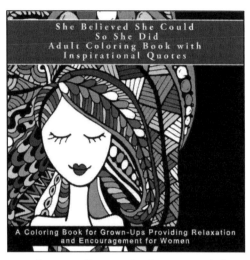

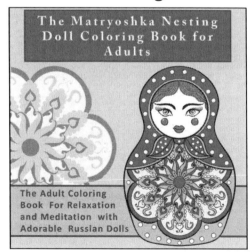

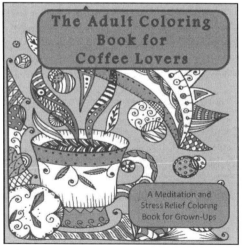

37944715R10059

Printed in Great Britain
by Amazon